No Hogwash
Diabetes

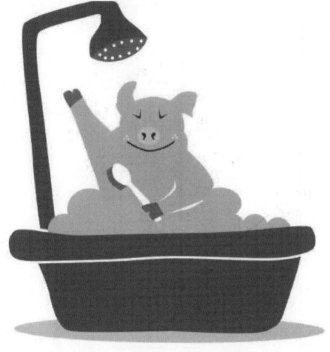

Natural Healing

By: Michael Von Irvin, MBA, BSN, RN

It is not the strongest of the species that survives, not the most
intelligent that survives. It is the one that is the most adaptable to
change.
—Charles Darwin

Testimonials
For Michael Von Irvin

To work with Michael Von Irvin or make comments contact
help@writersprofitguide.com

Michael

"My pleasure to add a distinguished professional, such as yourself, to my circle of friends. All the best to you and your loved ones."

Father of Steve Job's Founder Of Apple Computers

John Jandali

Author • "America's #1 Marketing Wizard" •
• "The Deal Maker" • "Master Negotiator"

A lot of people are saying great things about Mike Von Irvin.

Former New York City Healthcare executive. Former VP of AlphaCare and Director of Marketing for MLTC Consulting. Serial Entrepreneur.

Past appearances with Geraldo Rivera, Thomas Mesereau (Michael Jackson's Attorney), Tracy Morgan, Prince Royce, Rafael Furcal and many other celebrities, politicians, and sports stars.

BRANDING–My friend marketing whiz Michael Von Irvin says branding is pointless without good Copywriting to back it up. I think he's right.

—David Garfinkel (copywriting legend)

John Fleck

Owner

Wanted to give a shout out to Michael Von Irvin. In one day his coaching and guidance has made a huge difference in the direction of my business.

—Brad Szollose with Michael Von Irvin.

My second business meeting in the city was with businessman, speaker and trainer Michael Von Irvin and his wife Bella.

Some of our clients have included large healthcare plans such as AlphaCare NY - now Magellan Health. Fitango - innovative patient engagement solutions help to reduce costly readmissions and improve outcomes - NY, Special Touch Homecare LHCSA NY, ASDC, MD's, Nurse Practitioner Groups, FESCO Fire Equipment Company Birmingham/Atlanta/International, Irvin Brother's World Imports, IFPA - International Fire Protection Academy, Hood Master, Southern Fire Solutions, NAFFCO - Dubai, Exit Logic, Jessup Mfg - Chicago, MeridianRx (PBM) - Detroit, and other Healthcare Plans, Providers, Clarity, Tyco, SimplexGrinnell, FireMaster, Clinical, IT, Businesses, Marketing Related Companies, US Military Iraq.

To work with Michael Von Irvin or make comments contact
help@writersprofitguide.com

Introduction

This book is not meant to be a masterpiece of grammar. There may be grammatical mistakes. In the spirit of No Hogwash Books, we just try to get straight to the point and to hammer these points home. We are honored that you chose this book to read and study.

REMEMBER: It is what you get out of a book that is important. This book is not meant to cover all portions of the subject. It is meant to help you. In order to learn more and grow more we also have courses designed for each subject of interest.

Thanks so much. We are very grateful to consider you a friend.

For more info visit www.michaelvonirvin.com
Or www.nohogwashbooks.com

To work with Michael Von Irvin or make comments contact
help@writersprofitguide.com

If you are going to make a real change for the better, it will not be easy at first. And know this…..there are a lot of people who are looking out for your best interest. However, there are also a lot of people who will try to control you. I had to break free of negative people and learn how to live my life to the fullest.

- **Michael Von Irvin**

Thank you for purchasing this eBook.

Sign up for my FREE eNewsletter and receive special offers, access to bonus content, and info on the latest new releases and other great eBooks from Michael Von Irvin

at www.michaelvonirvin.com

To work with Michael Von Irvin or make comments contact
help@writersprofitguide.com

No Hogwash

Take Charge of Your

Diabetes

And Your Health

By: Michael Von Irvin, MBA, BSN, RN

Michael Von Irvin is an internationally recognized as health expert, marketing expert, businessman, and author who has helped others earn millions of dollars and develop great health. He has helped people in just about every business category turn their ideas into fortunes. Michael's No Hogwash approach is straight forward and aims to cut through the hype found in typical business and health related world. His knowledge has been given and accepted by successful people throughout the world. He started the No Hogwash Series in order to give straight forward information without the hype. For more money making and marketing and help tips and techniques, tactics, and strategies, go to www.michaelvonirvin.com or www.nohogwashbooks.com

To work with Michael Von Irvin or make comments contact
help@writersprofitguide.com

Table of Contents

Disclaimer

Nothing in this book should be construed to be medical advice or even the advice of a nutritionist or dietician. All of the comments herein are from personal experience. The author is absolved from any responsibility regarding any results from those who carry out the suggestions related in this book. Each reader is responsible for his or her own actions.

Introduction

So what's the big deal about diabetes? Hasn't diabetes always been around? Why so much emphasis on this disease in recent years? If these are questions you've been asking you'll be glad to know they will be answered in *The No Hogwash Approach to Understanding Diabetes.*

The difficulty regarding diabetes is two-fold. First is how insidious the disease actually is, and second is the ignorance and misunderstanding of the disease by the general public. It's this ignorance that is, in part, causing the growing epidemic not only in America, but literally around the world.

When surveys are done regarding how people rate the severity of health problems (i.e. cancer, heart disease, and diabetes), without fail, diabetes is listed far below the others – almost at the bottom of the list.

Why is this so? It's because you seldom, if ever, hear of someone dying from diabetes. Quite the opposite from cancer and heart disease. Generally, diabetes is thought of as a minor disease that is treatable. Available information tells us that with the right lifestyle changes, and the right medications, diabetes can be *controlled* and that the person with the disease can then live a *normal* life. So the question again is, what's the big deal?

Perception vs. Reality

This perception is light years from the reality of the situation. In truth, diabetes is a silent killer. Diabetes attacks the entire body affecting nearly every area. It is the leading cause of blindness, amputations, and kidney failure, and it can triple the risk for heart attack and stroke. With this in mind, here are a few statistics which substantiates the seriousness of this disease:

- *25.8 million Americans have diabetes — 8.3 percent of the U.S. population. Of these, 7 million do not know they have the disease.*
- *In 2010, about 1.9 million people ages 20 or older were diagnosed with diabetes.*

- *The number of people diagnosed with diabetes has risen from 1.5 million in 1958 to 18.8 million in 2010, an increase of epidemic proportions.*
- *It is estimated that 79 million adults aged 20 and older have prediabetes. Prediabetes is a condition where blood glucose levels are higher than normal but not high enough to be called diabetes.*

http://ndep.nih.gov/diabetes-facts/

Even with these frightening numbers glaring at us, the most ironic aspect is that diabetes is probably one of the most *preventable* diseases there is. It is almost totally what is known as a *lifestyle* disease.

Come along through this book and learn more details about diabetes, because to be well informed could save your life. This is a subject in which ignorance will never be *bliss.*

Chapter 1

What is Diabetes?

Who is Responsible for Your Health?

In generations past, our forebears seldom if ever went to the doctor. Oftentimes a doctor was miles away. Or there was none at all. Health care as we know it today was unheard of. Of course one could say this was both good and bad. Certainly modern medical discoveries have saved millions of lives. On the flip side, people who lived in those earlier times were well versed in natural medicines and medical treatments. In other words, by necessity they were responsible for their own well being.

In our present society we have moved poles apart from this mindset. The majority of people rely solely on doctors, prescriptions, and hospitals for their *health care*. In reality it has little to do with health care since it is primarily *illness care*.

To work with Michael Von Irvin or make comments contact
help@writersprofitguide.com

Few people know or understand the illnesses, diseases, or conditions that plague them. Instead they simply rely on a medical practitioner to *make them well* again. The problem is they were probably never *well* to begin with. At least not in the fullest sense of the word.

Learn to be Proactive

Compounding this problem is the fact that few if any of our trained physicians study *health.* Instead they train by studying *sickness, illness, and disease.* This is yet another reason why each and every individual must be responsible for his or her own health and well being. This is not to say one should ignore doctors or their advice. It is to say that you must be proactive in your own search for optimum health.

In order to move past a state of illness, one must have a clear concept of where they desire to be. One must decide "Do I want to control a disease? Or do I want to be whole, well, and healthy?" The choice is yours.

Optimum Health Defined

Over sixty years ago the World Health Organization created a definition of optimal health. It is "a state of complete physical, mental, and social well-being." This would mean that a truly healthy person focuses on healthcare as incorporating good nutrition, clean habits, sleep, exercise, relaxation and a social support system. For instance, a person who is disease-free, but is hooked on sleeping tablets can hardly be thought of has enjoying optimum health.

The core message of *The No Hogwash Approach to Understanding Diabetes* is that every person must become responsible for his or her own health – and healthcare. With that in mind, as we broach the subject of diabetes, the first step will be to dig down and learn what this condition truly is. What causes it? Why are some people prone to have these symptoms and others are not? Is there something more than medication that the sufferer can do about it? If you are serious about moving past where you are now, and moving toward enjoying optimum health, you will want to know this information.

To work with Michael Von Irvin or make comments contact
help@writersprofitguide.com

What is Diabetes?

The short definition tells us that diabetes is *a polygenic disease characterized by abnormally high glucose levels in the blood; any of several metabolic disorders marked by excessive urination and persistent thirst.*

A more detailed definition describes diabetes as the *presence of constant high blood sugar levels. In your body, the hormone insulin is used to take glucose (a type of sugar) from your bloodstream and put in into your fat, liver and muscle cells. When your body stops producing enough insulin to carry out this process, or when your cells stop responding to the insulin, the amount of sugar in your blood remains elevated.*

From these two definitions we see that glucose, or sugar, plays an important role in this disease. In fact, previous generations called it *sugar diabetes.* This was the name by which most people knew it. The connection is unmistakable.

However, this doesn't mean that every person who eats a lot of sugar and sweets has, or will have in the future, full-blown diabetes. It *does* mean that each one of us must understand the clear dangers of poor nutrition, and bad eating habits.

Types of Diabetes

Now that we have a better grasp of exactly what diabetes is, let's look at the different types.

There are two major types of diabetes: Type 1 and Type 2. Both Type 1 and Type 2 diabetes cause blood sugar levels to become higher than normal. However, they do this in different ways.

*• **Type 1 diabetes** (formerly called insulin-dependent diabetes or juvenile diabetes) is an autoimmune disease which occurs when the child's immune system starts to destroy its own insulin-producing cells in the pancreas. Because the pancreas is not able to produce insulin, children with type 1 diabetes need insulin to help keep their blood sugar levels within a normal range.*

- ***Type 2 diabetes*** *(formerly called non-insulin-dependent diabetes or adult-onset diabetes) is different. In contrast to someone with Type 1 diabetes, someone with Type 2 diabetes still produces insulin. But the body doesn't respond to the insulin normally. Excess weight and obesity can cause the insulin to not work correctly. When the insulin does not work correctly, glucose is less able to enter the cells and do its job of supplying energy (doctors call this insulin resistance). This causes the blood sugar level to rise, making the pancreas produce even more insulin. Eventually, the pancreas can wear out from working overtime to produce extra insulin. Then, the pancreas may no longer be able to produce enough insulin to keep a person's blood sugar levels within a normal range.*

For the purposes of this book, we will not be discussing Type 1 diabetes mellitus. Instead, we will focus on Type 2, as they are both quite different.

For many years, Type 2 diabetes was known as adult-onset diabetes mellitus (AODM). This name can no longer be applied since the age at which people develop this type of diabetes is dropping steadily. Today, children and teens are afflicted with this formerly adult-only disease. This is due mainly to poor eating habits, lack of quality nutrition, lack of exercise, and the resulting obesity.

Factors in Diabetes

It is true that some of the risk factors for Type 2 diabetes are out of your control.

- One might be genetics – perhaps there is a family tendency toward diabetes.
- Race may also play a part since people of certain races have a higher propensity toward this disease.
- The conditions present while you were forming in your mother's womb can also play a part in your genetic makeup.

• Aging also plays a part in the risk factors of diabetes.

None of the above means your fate is sealed – that you will surely be a victim of this disease. It simply means there will be a greater risk. The good news is there are risk factors that are totally within your control to change.

- Excess overall weight
- Excess weight around your middle
- Couch Potato Lifestyle – lack of exercise
- Poor diet – one that is high in saturated fats and sugar intake.

I think this is worth understanding, because type 2 diabetes is one of the few lifestyle disorders where 1) the basic causes are fairly well understood, and 2) we have effective diet/lifestyle prevention strategies that have been clearly proven by multiple controlled trials.

In Chapter 2, we'll see how the medical world deals with this disease of diabetes.

Chapter 2
How the Medical World Treats Diabetes
False Sense of Security

As mentioned in the previous chapter, we as a society have gotten lazy when it comes to self-discipline to attain a healthy body. It's so much easier to take a pill to lower cholesterol, for instance, than it is to change a lifestyle to lower cholesterol. Unfortunately, looking for good numbers (such as measuring cholesterol levels) does not equate optimum health, because the root problem has not been addressed.

The same is true with diabetes. Controlling blood sugar with medication will not get rid of the diabetes. In fact, what often happens is that the *normal numbers* lull the patient into a false sense of security which can then lead to even more neglect in personal proactive healthcare. How much better it would be to achieve the normal numbers (such as normal blood sugar) through a healthy diet and lifestyle changes.

To work with Michael Von Irvin or make comments contact
help@writersprofitguide.com

Treats Cause or Symptoms

In today's medical world, if a patient comes in with a severe injury, such as broken bones, lacerations, concussions, the treatment procedure works well. The extent of the injuries is ascertained and treatment quickly follows. As to the treatment, it matters little if the patient was in a car wreck, or fell from a two-story window. The cause does not affect the treatment of the resulting injuries.

When it comes to illnesses and disease, this system often fails the patient who is suffering from the symptoms. Contrary to an injury that may have occurred minutes before, an illness usually doesn't just appear overnight. While the symptoms may seem to have appeared overnight, the truth is hidden symptoms have been in place for months – perhaps even years. And what has taken years to develop will not disappear quickly.

For instance a patient displays high blood sugar – but not high enough to be full-blown diabetes. In most instances, it will not be considered *treatable* by the medical world until the numbers are higher. In other words, until it becomes a full-blown disease. A certain number-count will determine the treatment to be received. Little or no attention is paid to the lifestyle or diet of the patient. Manipulating numbers with medication only masks a disease. It does not equate to good health.

Studies clearly show that people with prediabetes may never get diabetes; nevertheless, they are still at severe risk. The fact is prediabetes actually isn't *pre-anything*. In and of itself it is known to be a serious health condition and thereby should be treated as early as possible.

To work with Michael Von Irvin or make comments contact
help@writersprofitguide.com

Exorbitant Cost of Diabetes

Treating the *causes* of diabetes – or prediabetes –
leads to a healthy individual. This is a person who is not
satisfied with simply masking symptoms. The desire to be
healthy can be a very strong motivator. However, there is yet
another motivator and that is the high cost of being sick.
Medical costs are exorbitant in the United States and diabetes
is quickly becoming one of the most expensive of all
illnesses.

*According to a 2007 study, "Economic Costs of Diabetes
in the U.S.," by the American Diabetes Association,
the cost of diabetes is even higher: $174 billion ($116
billion in total medical expenditures,
including drugs and office visits, in addition to the
hospital costs, and $58 billion in reduced national
productivity).*

- *One of every five health care dollars is spent caring
for someone with diabetes.*
- *Diabetics have medical expenditures that are 2.3
times higher than other victims of chronic disease.*
- *They have more frequent and longer hospital stays,
more doctor and emergency visits, more nursing facility*

stays, more home health visits, and more prescription drug and medical supply use.

> *Add to this the costs of the hidden diabetes epidemic: $18 billion for the estimated 6.3 million people with undiagnosed diabetes, and $25 billion for 57 million, or one in four, American adults with pre-diabetes. Those with pre-diabetes are likely to develop Type 2 diabetes within 10 years. If the current trend continues, one in three children faces a life with diabetes.*
>
> http://www.thefiscaltimes.com/Articles/ 2010/08/19/The-Cost-of-Diabetes

Yet another source puts the numbers into an even clearer perspective:

> *The American Diabetes Association (Association) released new research on March 6, 2013 estimating the total costs of diagnosed diabetes have risen to $245 billion in 2012 from $174 billion in 2007, when the cost was last examined.*

To bring this down to a more personal scale, the supplies needed to control this disease can often cost an individual several hundred dollars a month. Even with fairly good insurance coverage, there is still a lot of out-of-pocket expense.

And yet, it must be stated again that diabetes is one of the most preventable of all chronic diseases. It is without a doubt a lifestyle disease. We know this simply from how the epidemic has spread around the world with the influx of Western diets and lifestyles. For instance, India at one time had an extremely low rate of the diabetes. In more recent years their economy has begun to flourish; they now have a middle-class citizenry which is something new. Fast food restaurants flourish. More people are driving rather than walking. Long hours are being spent in an office where there is little or no exercise. Today diabetes is at or near epidemic numbers in India.

This is only one example of how the disease follows the lifestyle, which substantiates the premise that a change in lifestyle can also bring an individual back into a state of optimum health.

At the first of the chapter an example was given of a physical injury and I stated that the *cause* of the injury was of small importance in the treatment of the patient. Whether the patient was in a car wreck, or fell from a two-story window, the cause will not affect the treatment.

In dealing with disease, on the other hand, the *cause is of utmost importance* in treatment.

Prediabetes often means there are underlying metabolic imbalances. The successful treatment will not be focused on a disease, but rather to *remove* the things in that person's life that alters or damages metabolism. Further, it will focus on *providing* those things that enhance, optimize, and normalize the body's functioning. Better to treat the body's system rather than try to mask the symptom. It's better to treat an individual rather than treat a disease.

In order to fully appreciate what it means to treat the system, let's look at how our bodies truly function.

To work with Michael Von Irvin or make comments contact
help@writersprofitguide.com

Chapter 3

How the Body Works

It's a given that knowledge is power. This is especially true when it comes to knowing how our bodies work. The more we know about how the body functions and what it needs to function at highest efficiency, the more equipped we are to properly care for our bodies.

This could be compared to making the purchase of a brand new luxury import car. It's a sure bet that such an investment would cause the new owner to at least read the manual to see how things work and how such a car should be maintained. It's the same with the human body. (Or it should be.)

The problem is, not only do we not know how our bodies work, we neglect the even the most minimal care that is required. Past that, we then abuse our bodies with improper diet, lack of good nutrition, high levels of stress, lack of proper rest, and lack of necessary exercise. With this kind of treatment, we inadvertently set ourselves up for the onslaught of sickness, illness, and disease.

It Begins with Glucose

We'll begin by looking at an amazing substance known as glucose. All of the muscle cells and tissues of organs throughout your body rely on glucose for energy to function. Blood sugar actually is not the bad guy. It's rather like the rocket fuel for your body. Your body is so smart that it knows to store this glucose and then release it at the exact moment when it's needed the most. Problems arise when the glucose levels rise too high.

So where does this glucose come from? This power fuel comes from foods like fruits, vegetables, grains, and sugars from which your body then converts to tiny little sugar molecules we call glucose. Essentially it doesn't matter if you eat a piece of chocolate cake, or a plate full of broccoli, all carbohydrate foods contain chains of sugar molecules.

To work with Michael Von Irvin or make comments contact
help@writersprofitguide.com

Once the food is eaten the digestive enzymes break the food down for use in the body. When broken apart the chains are converted into glucose, fructose, or galactose. However, there is one more stop along the way to the cells of your body and that is the liver. It is in the liver where the extra glucose is stored for later use. (When stored in the liver it is in the form of glycogen.) Now the glucose is ready to get going to provide power and energy to your mind, muscles, and metabolism.

Now you may be thinking that if all carbohydrates convert to glucose, then it makes little difference what foods are eaten. Right? Wrong! The big difference is in the simple matter of how much time – or how little time – it takes for the food to be digested. For instance foods that rank high in the glycemic index (more about the glycemic index later in the book), such as white rice, white bread, and processed foods are digested quickly, absorbed quickly and then cause a spike in blood sugar.

On the other hand, foods that rank lower on the glycemic index move through the digestive system more slowly and thereby sugar (glucose) is released into the body slowly. For instance a carb that is surrounded by a protective coating, such as beans and seeds, takes longer to move through the digestive system. Oatmeal, lentils, whole grain cereals and grain products are also in this category.

So far, so good. We know what glucose is and how the body uses it. We also know how crucial glucose is for the body to function as it was designed to function. Now we'll take a look at what causes things to malfunction.

Toxic Glucose

As necessary as glucose is, if it's just floating around in your bloodstream it becomes toxic to the body. But once again, your body is so smart, it has an incredible defense mechanism set in place. Any glucose that is not immediately used is stored as glycogen in the liver and the muscles.

To work with Michael Von Irvin or make comments contact
help@writersprofitguide.com

This wouldn't be such a problem except for the fact that your body has only a limited number of glycogen receptors. When these receptors are full – and they nearly always are in the body of an overweight, inactive individual – the body is left with only one option. Now it must store all the excess glucose as saturated fat within the body. This is the first step in the malfunction.

If that expensive car we talked about earlier had an oil leak, and that oil leak was ignored, it could affect yet another part in the car, and then another, which would cause the problems to escalate. It's the same with your body.

Eventually, when the body senses glucose in the bloodstream, now the pancreas is put on the alert. It's the job of beta cells in the pancreas to releases a hormone called *insulin*. The insulin then signals the body to store the glucose as glycogen. These smart cells are designed to sense glucose levels in the bloodstream and adjust insulin output accordingly.

If the glycogen receptors are full and it can't do this, the body thinks that the cells didn't get the message. It's like the body is calling out, "Are you awake out there? I said I need more insulin." The pancreas hears the call and then responds by releasing even more insulin.

Now let's say this pattern is repeated on a daily basis, which it obviously is in the overweight or inactive person who lives on fatty and sugary foods.

The cells are getting an overdose of insulin, so they eventually become resistant to the very presence of insulin. (Ever hear of insulin resistance?) The scene is now set for the perfect vicious cycle. Round and round it goes.

To work with Michael Von Irvin or make comments contact
help@writersprofitguide.com

The body is now getting desperate. The pancreas releases even more insulin, trying to get the cells to uptake the toxic glucose. Excess insulin in the bloodstream is also toxic. So now we have toxic excessive glucose, and toxic excessive insulin. What happens next? All of this works to damage the receptors on these cells. The beta cells are slowly losing their smart ability to sense changes in blood sugar levels. They are no longer producing the right amount at the right time. Blood sugars will now rise – sometimes to dangerous levels. The well-tuned machine is beginning to malfunction just the same as if you put sugar in the gas tank of your expensive car.

Eventually, the insulin just sort of gives up. Unable to do its job properly it is now forced to allow the glucose access to your fat cells just to get it out of the bloodstream. So now you can see that fat isn't stored as fat in the body. Rather *sugar* (from carbohydrates) is stored as fat. This is probably quite different than most people might have imagined regarding weight gain.

Tuning Up Your Machine

That toxic glucose that is pulsing around in your body wondering where to go, can be taken care of quite easily by a structured exercise program. As your muscles contract and relax during exercise, they are taking in more and more glucose from the bloodstream and putting it to work in the form of energy.

Remember those *deaf* cells that became resistant to insulin? Exercise can take care of that problem as well. Studies have shown that exercise causes the muscles cells to become more sensitive to signals from insulin. It's as though muscles cells fall asleep when not in use and proteins that usually accept glucose and convert it to energy become less and less active.

This is why the experts in the field of wellness repeatedly contend that diabetes is one of the most preventable – and yes even reversible – of all the chronic diseases.

In this chapter we've seen how problems begin in the body, now it's time to see what happens when problems escalate.

To work with Michael Von Irvin or make comments contact
help@writersprofitguide.com

Chapter 4
How Problems Escalate

In Chapter 3 we learned exactly how an overabundance of glucose in the body happens. We also learned that this excess of glucose in turn causes an excess of insulin. In this chapter we will follow this unhealthy, and quite dangerous, progression.

Once the cells have become insulin resistant, the beta cells in the pancreas (sensing this rise in glucose) compensate by producing even more insulin. These body cells are no longer responding to that "key" that the insulin once effectively used to "unlock the door" which would allow the glucose to come in and be converted to energy. In the early stages of this *condition* the individual may very well still have normal blood glucose levels.

Those who have insulin resistance may manage to show normal blood glucose levels, but the body is beginning to malfunction. In fact, the body does not like all that circulating insulin so it begins to compensate in ways that may for a time be completely hidden.

- Triglyceride levels rise. Triglycerides are a type of fat found in your blood. Your body uses them for energy.

Some triglycerides are necessary for good health; however, high levels of triglycerides can raise the risk of heart disease and may be a sign of *metabolic syndrome.*

- HDL cholesterol (good cholesterol) drops. We know that the higher the HDL cholesterol levels, the lower the risk of heart disease.

- The body retains sodium. This relates to the well-known adage: "For every action, there is a reaction." This is true of high insulin levels – it causes sodium retention which in turn raises blood pressure.

- There can also be a rise in blood pressure apart from sodium intake. This means that there is a problem with high blood pressure for reasons other than sodium retention.

- Blood-clotting factors – such as fibrinogen – go into overdrive. Eventually, these can cause tiny blood clots that will eventually clog arteries.

- LDL cholesterol (known as the *bad* cholesterol) particles become too dense.

To work with Michael Von Irvin or make comments contact
help@writersprofitguide.com

This in turn increases the risk of heart problems.

The list above is why diabetes has been called the *silent killer*. These complications are working together until eventually one day the hidden becomes very obvious and all sorts of symptoms begin to manifest. Now the body is one step closer to Type 2 diabetes (*impaired glucose tolerance*).

Glucose Intolerance

When insulin is not working properly, it is no longer able to guide the glucose (or sugar) into the proper cells. Now the glucose must stay in the bloodstream which raises blood sugar. When this happens consistently, day in and day out, the high blood sugar begins to cause damage to the eyes, kidneys, nerves, and blood vessels.

Prediabetes vs. Metabolic Syndrome

There is often confusion between prediabetes and metabolic syndrome – both of which may be precursors to diabetes. Pre-diabetes is diagnosed by mildly elevated blood glucose levels (hyperglycemia). You do not have to have any other symptoms to be diagnosed with prediabetes.

Metabolic syndrome on the other hand will be diagnosed by evidence of several different symptoms such as:

- Obesity
- High cholesterol
- High blood pressure
- High blood sugar level

As you can see being diagnosed with prediabetes does not mean you have metabolic syndrome. However, if you are diagnosed with metabolic syndrome, you will definitely have prediabetes.

Full Blown Diabetes

At some point in this slow-moving continuum, the individual will no doubt end up in the doctor's office. What are they looking for? Answers to why they are suffering from the symptoms. And what do most patients want? A quick fix to make them *well*. Or to help *control* their newly-diagnosed disease of diabetes.

To work with Michael Von Irvin or make comments contact
help@writersprofitguide.com

By this point the vicious cycle has become even more vicious. Now the beta cells in the pancreas can no longer produce enough insulin, thus the blood glucose levels are free to rise even higher.

Let's take an even closer look at what is happening here. As long as sufficient insulin is being produced the body sensors get the message that there is enough energy available to keep on living. But, when the pancreas can no longer produce sufficient insulin, the body panics and cries out: "Oh no, we're short on energy." Now the liver hears the cry for help and kicks in to do its part. What does it do? It releases the extra stores of glucose. Of course this only compounds the problem – because now the blood glucose levels are shooting even higher.

As you can see, our bodies are highly complex, finely tuned machines. Every part is connected to another part. Nothing stands alone, or operates alone. This is why when things goes wrong, such as glucose intolerance, and we treat that one symptom, it fails to take into account the root cause of the problem that begins way back with diet and lifestyle.

As mentioned earlier, most people rate heart disease above diabetes in the level of a dangerous disease. They have no idea that very often it is the diabetes, or prediabetes, that is the root cause of heart disease.

To work with Michael Von Irvin or make comments contact
help@writersprofitguide.com

Chapter 5
Diabetes and the Heart

Damage to Blood Vessels

In the last chapter it was mentioned that glucose intolerance can damage blood vessels. The person who has little knowledge of how the body works may never make the connection between the condition of diabetes and the condition of heart trouble. But, because the body systems are all intricately connected with one another, there is a very real and very serious connection.

Your heart and blood vessels make up your circulatory system. Your heart is an amazing muscle that pumps blood through your body. The heart pumps blood carrying oxygen to large blood vessels, called arteries, and small blood vessels, called capillaries. Other blood vessels, called veins, carry blood back to the heart.

High blood sugars in the bloodstream over time will create inflammation in the blood vessels. Inflammation can lead to cracks and lesions in the blood vessel walls, which then is repaired with a substance called low-density lipoprotein (LDL) cholesterol.

You've probably heard of LDL. Your doctor tests your LDL levels when you get your cholesterol checked. You may have heard him refer to LDL as your "bad" cholesterol. This label is not entirely true.

Actually, LDL fulfills several important roles in the body. This includes tissue and vessel wall repair, hormone production, insulation of nerves, and proper brain function. If high blood sugar has damaged your blood vessel walls, your smart liver will manufacture LDL to repair that damage. Because LDL is a sticky substance, it will then collect unhealthy trans-fatty acids and calcium. This condition, over time may lead to a blockage in the blood vessel.

This damage begins with the very smallest of blood vessels – the capillaries. High concentrations of glucose cause weakness in the walls. Once weakened the vessels have a tendency to burst. When they burst, the body (smart as it is) now creates a scar tissue as it works to heal – this scar tissue, in turn, can actually then damage the organs which those vessels serve.

To work with Michael Von Irvin or make comments contact
help@writersprofitguide.com

If this is not problematic enough – it tends to worsen. LDL cholesterol is susceptible to damage by oxygen-free radicals. When the LDL particles cling to the artery walls, they work almost like magnets for these free radicals. As the free radicals attack the LDL particles the plaque surface becomes rough and uneven. This process further narrows the vessels.

The smart liver has a very sophisticated way to filter out excess LDL particles. The liver is designed to grab LDL particles, corral them, and send them out through the digestive tract. The problem is Type 2 diabetes greatly impairs this amazing filtering system.

Perhaps you can now understand how diabetes and heart problems are so closely intertwined. This list below gives even more insight:

As many as 65% of people diagnosed with diabetes will eventually die of a heart attack or a stroke. Diabetes greatly increases the risk of a heart attack or a stroke in the following ways:

- *By speeding up the process where the walls of the artery malfunction and they get clogged inside (arteriosclerosis)*

- *By altering blood cholesterol and fat levels*

- *By making the blood more prone to clotting*

http://www.netwellness.org/healthtopics/diabetes/faq3.cfm

Damaged blood vessels could affect the eyes (blindness), the brain (stroke), feet (requiring amputation of toe, foot, or in extreme cases the entire leg).

What are some of the things that cause damaged blood vessels?

- High blood sugar (over a long period of time)
- High cholesterol (other abnormal blood fats)
- High blood pressure
- Use of tobacco
- Diet of too much saturated fat
- Obesity
- Sedentary lifestyle

Now that you understand more clearly how diabetes and prediabetes are so closely connected, in the next chapter we'll discuss what obesity has to do with diabetes.

To work with Michael Von Irvin or make comments contact
help@writersprofitguide.com

Chapter 6
Diabetes and Obesity

Weight-Loss Programs

The subject of *weight loss* has become so prevalent in our society, it's generally ignored. There are weight loss pills, fad diets, and even weight loss equipment. Add to that the books and literature explaining exactly how to lose weight. All of this equates out to millions of dollars spent, and yet the majority of Americans are still overweight.

According to a 2006 study reported in *The New England Journal of Medicine*, most people who participate in weight-loss programs "regain about one-third of the weight lost during the next year and are typically back to baseline in three to five years."

http://www.businessweek.com/debateroom/archives/2008/01/the_diet_indust.html

We have become an inactive, sedentary, comfort-seeking generation. We love to eat and we love to eat what we want to eat. Little thought goes into what the body is battling just because we felt we deserved that *baconator*. Or that second can of sugary soda pop. Or the last of the chocolate cake right before bedtime. (It was just sitting there in the fridge calling your name.)

But as we have seen in the previous chapters, no matter what we choose to ingest, the faithful, hardworking, extremely smart body goes into double time in order to do its level best to correctly process all of that extra fat and high levels of sugar. And it will do so until it can do so no longer – whether that end result is a full-blown case of Type 2 diabetes, or high blood pressure, or heart attack, or stroke.

Diabesity

The correlation between obesity and diabetes is now so well documented that the medical world has coined the term *diabesity*.

To work with Michael Von Irvin or make comments contact
help@writersprofitguide.com

Diabesity is the continuum of metabolic disturbances from mild blood sugar and insulin imbalances to pre-diabetes to full blown type 2 diabetes. It occurs in about 40% of people of normal weight – these are the skinny fat people who look thin but are metabolically fat and have all the same risk factors for disease and death as those who are overweight. And it occurs in 80% of overweight people.

http://www.doctoroz.com/videos/diabesity-reversible-epidemic

These are statistics that no one can afford to ignore. The truth is, diabesity is a condition that is the result of social, economic and political conditions. Obesity and diabetes are social diseases. It bears little or no resemblance to the diseases that plagued our ancestors, many of which were diseases carried by insects, rats, or the spread of germs.

It's a sad indictment of our nation (and much of the world) that children under the age of ten are now getting Type 2 diabetes (what used to be called adult onset). We are seeing strokes and heart attacks in people as young as fifteen or twenty. Unless we begin to make drastic changes, in a few years one in three children born today will eventually have diabetes.

Excess Weight and Prediabetes

Let's see how that excess weight heightens the prediabetes condition. Increased insulin levels can lead to an out-of-control appetite. This then leads to increased weight gain around the belly, added inflammation and oxidative stress, and myriad other effects: high blood pressure; high cholesterol; low HDL, high triglycerides; thickening of the blood; and increased risk of cancer, Alzheimer's, and depression.

Carrying around extra weight can be compared to pressing your finger over the end of the water hose when it's going full blast. It causes the water to come out at an increased pressure. It also causes pressure within the hose itself. This is what happens to blood vessels when the size of the opening decreases.

Those who are overweight put that type of pressure on their heart and the blood vessels. They expect their heart to pump hard enough to get blood to all of the excess tissue hour after hour, day after day. This is in spite of the fact that many of the veins and arteries are clogged due to the causes described in the previous chapter.

To work with Michael Von Irvin or make comments contact
help@writersprofitguide.com

Fat around the midsection reacts differently from fat in other parts of the body. These central fat cells release more free fatty acids. The increased number of free fatty acids cause what is known as *vascular reactivity*. This means the blood vessels are now contracting more than they were designed to contract. The end result is high blood pressure. (Just like the finger over the end of the water hose.)

Slow Process of Weight Gain

Extra pounds have a way of sneaking up on you. All of a sudden those favorite slacks, or that favorite skirt, is thrown to the back of the closet. The tight fit is just too uncomfortable. But you're sure you'll be digging it back out as soon as you get back on that diet you started last month. This is to say, the problem is never really taken seriously. There are far too many other pressing things on your daily agenda. The busyness of your life means another skipped breakfast, another fast food lunch, another shot of caffeine, another late dinner created from processed foods filled with additives and chemicals. Your body deserves better.

The purpose of this book is to help you to awaken to the fact that danger signals such as weight gain should not be ignored. Your body is speaking to you. It's time to make the decision to listen.

Getting Serious

In our society, weight loss has been equated with looking good. The diet pills and fad diets never address the symptoms of prediabetes or hypertension. As long as we continue to think in this vein, we will never get serious about optimum health. Weight loss is about living a rich life that is full of vibrant health, high levels of energy, and a sense of well being. That's the quality effects of weight control – not how you look on the beach in a swimsuit.

The next chapter points to ways in which changes in eating habits can be life-saving.

To work with Michael Von Irvin or make comments contact
help@writersprofitguide.com

Chapter 7
Diabetes and Wrong Food Choices

The Manufacture of Food

We have already alluded to the fact that fatty, sugary, low-nutrient-density, empty-calorie food types pass through the digestive system rather quickly. There is little or no substance for the digestive system to work on. The faster the food passes through this system, the more quickly it spills into the blood system in the form of glucose.

One has only to take a quick look back at the history of civilization to grasp how far we've come in our desecration of what we call food. At one time people grew their food. Or raised the livestock and butchered their own meat. Or gathered roots, nuts and berries. Nowadays, food has become a manufacturing industry. In the laboratories and manufacturing plants where foods are "processed," the vital nutrients are removed and chemicals and additives are added in. All for the sake of long shelf life – and all for the sake of making a bigger and bigger profit.

It is the empty-calorie foods that have taken a massive toll on the vast majority of our population. The body is attempting to work with substances that have little more nutritional value than a plateful of sawdust. Sugary beverages play havoc with the liver and pancreas simply because the body is not designed for such a large intake of sugar.

Let's take a close look at what happens when a can of sweet soda pop is ingested. (This also applies to other sweets as well.)

Dopamine

One of the reasons why sweet foods have such an appeal to us is because they trigger the release of the feel-good chemical *dopamine*. Over a long period of time, it becomes another one of those vicious cycles mentioned earlier in the book. The more sugar we eat, the less dopamine produced by our brains. Why? It's because the constant intake of sugar eventually dulls the triggering effects. It literally wears down the brain's ability to produce dopamine. We develop a resistance.

To work with Michael Von Irvin or make comments contact
help@writersprofitguide.com

You may be thinking this might be a good thing if feel-good effects are no longer associated with our incessant "sweet tooth." In reality, what happens is similar to a drug habit – we continue to search for that great dopamine boost and can't find it. In our search, we just continue to shovel in the sweet cookies, candy, soda pop, and pastries. You can easily see how this can lead to overeating as we overcompensate to get that *feeling*.

Food in its Natural State

Let's return to the subject of how the diet of our ancestors differs from ours. Foods consumed in their most natural state contain high levels of nutrients that the body needs to function correctly. It also contains high levels of fiber, most of which is nonexistent in processed foods. For instance refined bleached white flour has had all of the fiber and nutritive values removed in the milling process. This process removes the outer layers of the grain where all the fiber and phytonutrients are concentrated. Again, this is so that there is no spoilage on the grocery shelf. By the time the manufacturer is finished, not even a grain weevil is interested. This is also true for the processing of rice, sugar, other grains – and many canned foods as well.

The Wonder of Fiber

Dr. Dennis Burkitt, a famous English physician, made a study of indigenous African bushmen and found that, for the most part, this people-group was free of conditions that plague our society — including heart disease, cancer, diabetes, and obesity. In his study he further discovered that the average hunter and gatherer ate 100 grams of fiber from all manner of roots, berries, leaves and plant foods. And the fiber is what helped our ancestors stay healthy as well. Compare that with the fact that the average American eats about 8 grams of fiber a day. Big difference.

There are many benefits to having a high amount of fiber in your daily diet. One of the most important is the fact that fiber cannot be digested quickly. It tends to stay in the gut for a longer period of time, hence it creates a sense of fullness. It lessens the tendency to grab a mid-morning or mid-afternoon sugary snack. The mind isn't thinking about a quick fix because the tummy is registering *full* to the brain.

If you're not sure how to begin introducing sufficient fiber into your diet, here are a few good suggestions:

To work with Michael Von Irvin or make comments contact
help@writersprofitguide.com

- *Get the flax. Get a coffee grinder just for flax seeds, grind 1/2 cup at a time, and keep in a tightly sealed glass jar in the fridge or freezer. Eat 2 tablespoons of ground flax seeds a day. Sprinkle on salads, grains, or vegetable dishes or mix in a little unsweetened applesauce.*
- *Load up on legumes. Beans beat out everything else for fiber content!*
- *Bulk up on vegetables. With low levels of calories and high levels of antioxidants and protective phytochemicals, these excellent fiber sources should be heaped on your plate daily.*
- *Go with the grain. Whole grains like brown rice or quinoa are rich in fiber, too.*
- *Eat more fruit. Include a few servings of low-sugar fruits to your diet daily (berries are the highest in fiber and other protective phytochemicals).*
- *Go nuts. Include a few handfuls of almonds, walnuts, pecans, or hazelnuts to your diet every day.*
- *Start slowly. Switching abruptly to a high-fiber diet can cause gas and bloating. Increase your fiber intake slowly until you get up to 50 grams a day.*

Glycemic Index

Fiber is one way to train your body to move away from empty calories to healthier foods that create a true sense of fullness. This is not a quick fix – not like a diet pill – but rather a lifestyle change that will stay with you for the rest of your life. Essentially, you are retaining your minds, emotions, and habits.

Yet another way to learn about nutritive value of food is to understand the glycemic index. This is how it works. This index measures how much a certain amount of food raises your blood-sugar levels. Foods that are high on the index scale tend to raise blood-sugar levels. Additionally, they cause an insulin spike. These foods that are high on the GI scale are quickly metabolized in the body which means you will be hungry again much sooner.

To work with Michael Von Irvin or make comments contact
help@writersprofitguide.com

To learn more about the Glycemic Index and how you can use it to begin to adjust your diet, run an online search. Many sites offer a full chart of which foods are either high or low on the index. Here's one that can get your started: *http://www.whfoods.com/genpage.php?tname=faq&dbid=32#where*

As you will soon see, the main focal point of a healthy diet is to consume foods in as near to their natural state as possible. Such foods are also referred to as *whole foods*. A snack of trail mix that contains nuts, seeds, and dried fruits is nutrient-rich, full of fiber, and much more filling than a glazed donut.

No More Cravings

What most people find, once they retrain their minds and bodies to eat healthy foods, is that the old harmful food cravings will slowly, but surely, disappear. This is because your body is reverting to its healthy state in which all of the systems described earlier in the book are functioning as they were designed.

Here are a few more reasons why whole foods help in disease prevention, and lead to optimum health

- *Foods rich in soluble fiber, such as oats, beans, and nuts, have been shown to lower LDL (bad) cholesterol significantly, not only in persons with high cholesterol, but even in healthy subjects.*

• *The fiber in a whole foods diet also lowers serum triglycerides, its potassium and magnesium drop blood pressure and its rich supply of antioxidants, such as vitamin E, protect cholesterol from free radical damage.*

• *The healthy polyunsaturated fats found in nuts significantly improve the quality of LDL cholesterol and body's ability to process and clear it.*

•*Diets rich in plant foods are also high in arginine, an essential amino acid that research is now beginning to focus on as an essential constituent of nitric oxide (NO). A vasodilator, NO relaxes blood vessels, improving blood flow.*

http://www.whfoods.com/genpage.php?tname=george&dbid=130

It's a sad fact that the majority of people who need to get healthy resist making the needed changes because they aren't ready to give up their comfort foods. Once again, this points to lack of understanding of what the body truly needs to function correctly. In the next chapter we'll see what part exercise plays in all of this.

To work with Michael Von Irvin or make comments contact
help@writersprofitguide.com

Chapter 8

Diabetes and Necessary Exercise

Mixed Signals

A healthy diet and exercise go hand-in-hand when it comes to dealing with obesity, prediabetes and diabetes. The reason most people fail to exercise and get moving is because they either don't have time, (at least they *think* they don't have time), or they simply believe that they *hate exercise.*

Again, our culture has given us many mixed signals when it comes to exercise. As with the idea of dieting, the main goals seems to be for looks alone. But the need for *movement* in the human body cannot be overemphasized. The human body is designed to work best when there is activity – movement.

It's time to stop thinking about looking good, or even *feeling good* when it comes to regular exercise. Instead, it's time to think about saving your own life. Or at least extending the years of your life. For those who suffer from diabetes or prediabetes, this is not something to be taken lightly. Let's look at a few specific areas in which exercise is beneficial.

Improves Blood Sugar

For many people their lives consist of getting out of the house and into the car, and then out of the car and into the workplace, and then back into the house to eat an evening meal. After that, it's an evening spent on the couch watching mindless television. Or hours browsing on the computer.

Intentional, regular, structured exercise greatly improves blood sugars. Muscles that are used are better able to make use of the insulin produced in the body. The movement literally increases *peripheral insulin sensitivity*. As was explained earlier, it is the insulin insensitivity that is problematic for a person who is diabetic.

Exercise produces increased glucose uptake in your muscles, and the effect can last for several hours. Interestingly enough, studies have proven that a single exercise session is able to improve insulin sensitivity in the liver and muscles for over sixteen hours.

Lowers Cardiovascular Risk Factors

Yet another wonderful benefit of exercise for the diabetic is that it works to lower blood pressure. Additionally, it raises the good cholesterol and decreases the triglycerides and the *bad* cholesterol.

Weight Loss

Even when weight loss is not the primary objective of a regular exercise program, inevitably the weight loss occurs. The pounds begin to drop as the body is put into motion on a regular basis.

"No Hogwash 111 Ways To Lose Weight Without Dieting" was written to help people lose weight without dieting. Available at Amazon books.

The Sense of Well Being

While most people may struggle to begin an exercise program, once it is underway, once it becomes a part of the daily routine, it begins to produce an unmistakable sense of well being. What happens is that the body begins to produce endorphins which are the natural body chemicals similar to opiates. The good feeling is also related to heightened mood levels. Endorphins also work as pain control, improve the immune system, and also improve the inflammatory response.

Choice of Exercise

Generally speaking, people who dread exercise make it way too complicated. They may think it has to be a membership at the local gym. Or buying all kinds of exercise equipment – and the fitness apparel to go with it. The fact is all you need is a good pair of walking shoes, and the determination to walk out the door and down the street.

Of course, if you love tennis, or swimming, or biking then by all means take that avenue. But walking is by far the simplest, easiest, cheapest and most readily accessible way in which to get started exercising.

To work with Michael Von Irvin or make comments contact
help@writersprofitguide.com

Start Small

If you are still a rookie at exercising, it would probably be best to begin with a fifteen-minute walk each day and gradually increase up to thirty. Also it's best to begin on flat areas, if that is possible. Save the hills for later on. This undertaking will require dedication and planning. Set a specific time for your daily walk and stick with it until it becomes an ingrained habit.

If weather is a problem where you live (in the cold North for instance) then join a group of local *mall walkers*. You can find them in nearly every community. They gather together to walk the malls before the shops open and customers arrive. It's yet another way to simplify your exercise program.

Beginners should start out slow and work up. And be sure to consult your doctor to see the best times of day to exercise. This will be especially important for an insulin-dependent diabetic.

In order to burn the most calories, be intentional about putting your whole body into each stride. Swing your arms as you walk. Some walkers like to bring their balled-up fist up to chest level and actually pump their arms much like a jogger or running would.

Your aim is to be invigorated but not exhausted. If you push too hard at the outset and overdo, then you will want to slack off the next day. That defeats the whole purpose.

As a guideline, you want to be breathing harder, but still be able to carry on a conversation. Create a rhythm that best suits you and your present energy levels and go with that.

As you progress each day, you will find that you are now looking forward to getting out and getting moving. Gradually your energy levels will rise, and each day you will feel the added strength.

To work with Michael Von Irvin or make comments contact
help@writersprofitguide.com

Stretch Out

Another important tip is to stretch before and after your walking routine. Stretch arms, calves, legs and torso. At first, even your stretches may feel stiff and awkward but after a few weeks, those muscles will become more flexible and you will feel more limber.

Pedometer

One great way to add a spark of motivation is to purchase a pedometer. This little device clips to your waistband and it measures your number of steps. Those who start using a pedometer create for themselves a step-goal and then strive to meet that goal and eventually exceed it.

Start by simply wearing the pedometer throughout the course of a several days – measuring your steps in a normal day. Once you know approximately how many steps are taken in a normal day, then begin to build on that number via your walking routine. Every 2,000 steps equal about a mile, and most people can walk one mile in about fifteen or twenty minutes. You can increase your steps if you make it a practice to walk during your lunch break in addition to your walking routine. Or find other ways throughout the day to increasingly bump up your steps to reach your goals.

Using Intervals

Another great way to keep fit with walking is to try introducing *intervals*. This should come later on after you've developed a good routine. As you speed up your pace somewhat you will burn more calories and you will become a faster walker. In other words increase your walk intensity for one minute, then slow for about five minute, then repeat. Try several variations of the interval-type walking. See what motivates you, and what invigorates you, and what challenges you.

Finding the Time

In our busy lives it's finding the time to exercise that becomes the most challenging. The trick is to get creative. Begin to look for down times that can be used for active movement. Where and when do you find yourself sitting and waiting? One soccer mom decided that instead of sitting in the stands during her son's games, she would get out and walk around the field. What about waiting at the bus stop? Instead of just standing there – or sitting –walk around and keep stretching your legs.

To work with Michael Von Irvin or make comments contact
help@writersprofitguide.com

Have you seen the small indoor exercise trampolines? What a great way to get your blood pumping – by jumping for a few minutes on the mini-tramp. Because they are small, you can do a workout while watching your favorite television show. Exercise balls are yet another way to get creative with indoor exercise.

For those who are reluctant to get out and walk – for whatever reason – try exercise videos and do your structured workout right there in your living room.

As you cast about for ideas and opportunities for exercise, soon you will realize that not having time is just an old worn-out excuse. One that is keeping you from enjoying a long, healthy life.

Even More Benefits

Those who look at weight loss in terms of a quick fix so they can drop a few pounds seldom if ever maintain that loss. However, those who begin to eat nutrient-rich foods (as described in the previous chapter), and then couple that change with regular exercise, are the ones whose lives are forever changed for the better. Nothing about such changes speaks of fads or even short-term solutions. Rather it is a complete change of lifestyle. It's there for the long-term.

Studies have shown that such changes have a powerful impact on blood sugar control. Some control programs showed that blood sugar counts fell three times lower for those who exercised than with those who simply *dieted*. This is because regular exercise helps the cells in the body to become more sensitive to insulin. And that's the results you are after!

Controlled blood sugar is a great reward for these lifestyle changes, but there are yet more benefits to regular exercise.

- Losing fat and gaining muscle means a slimmer physique.
- Increased muscle means metabolism speeds up
- Increased muscle creates strength and energy
- Exercise can be compared to taking antidepressant drugs (without the side effects). Mood levels are lifted.
- Weight-bearing exercise – like walking – also increases bone density.
- Regular exercise improves balance and reduces changes of falling.

To work with Michael Von Irvin or make comments contact
help@writersprofitguide.com

Now that you understand how crucial diet and exercise can be in the prevention and the reversing of diabetes, let's look at how stress can be a factor and what you can do about it.

Chapter 9

Diabetes and The Stress Factor

It doesn't take a genius to know that stress is harmful to your health in many ways, but did you know that stress is one of the factors in raising blood sugar levels?

The body is designed to handle short bursts of stress – especially when there is impending danger, or even when an exciting event is approaching. However, the body is *not* designed to handle ongoing stress and anxiety all day every day with no break or letup.

Our lives, just as in all of nature, should be in a rhythm pattern. The seasons change; the tides roll in and out; animals hibernate; the caterpillar spins a cocoon. People who run at high speed day after day often fool themselves into thinking this is way life has to be. That they have no choice. But that's not true. Your body, your mind, and your emotions need times of rest, relaxation, and play. And you are the only one who is in charge of creating those times of rest.

To work with Michael Von Irvin or make comments contact
help@writersprofitguide.com

It's time to get purposeful about controlling stress rather than simply being a victim of stress. Stress management is crucial for the diabetic or prediabetes-prone individual.

Understanding Cortisol

Cortisol is a key stress hormone that is secreted into the bloodstream and is responsible for several stress-related changes in the body. When the increases of cortisol are small it has good effects such as:

- A quick burst of energy for survival reasons
- Heightened memory functions
- A burst of increased immunity
- Lower sensitivity to pain
- Helps maintain homeostasis in the body

Stress Dangers

However, in our fast-paced society, cortisol levels are often too high and extend for long periods of time which then leads to an adverse effect. Many people are quite surprised to learn how dangerous ongoing stress can be. Take a look at some of the problems caused by excessive levels of cortisol:

- *Impaired cognitive performance*
- *Suppressed thyroid function*

- *Blood sugar imbalances such as hyperglycemia*
- *Decreased bone density*
- *Decrease in muscle tissue*
- *Higher blood pressure*
  - *Lowered immunity and inflammatory responses in the body, slowed wound healing, and other health consequences*
  - *Increased abdominal fat, which is associated with a greater amount of health problems than fat deposited in other areas of the body. Some of the health problems associated with increased stomach fat are heart attacks, strokes, the development of metabolic syndrome, higher levels of "bad" cholesterol (LDL) and lower levels of "good" cholesterol (HDL), which can lead to other health problems!*

http://stress.about.com/od/stresshealth/a/cortisol.htm

To work with Michael Von Irvin or make comments contact
help@writersprofitguide.com

If your goal is to achieve optimum health you will want to learn all you can about stress management. Entire books have been written about how to manage stress. Study, research, and take action steps.

Learn to be good to yourself. Give yourself time out even if it's only fifteen minutes a day. Get a massage. Try aromatherapy. Take a long soak in a bubble bath. Laugh a lot. Surround yourself with uplifting friends who support you and value you. Take time to do what you love to do, such as a hobby or avocation. Look for opportunities to do good things for others. Helping others helps you take your mind off your own cares and concerns. The list of how to de-stress is virtually endless.

Those who feel they are a helpless victim of constant stress are doomed to suffer. Granted there are stress factors over which we may have no control; but there are also many stress factors that we *can*control. We *have control* over how we respond to a traffic jam, for instance. View it as a great opportunity to practice meditation, or deep breathing exercises. It becomes your choice to turn off the stress and turn on the relaxation techniques. Incorporate as many as you possibly can in the course of a day.

Self-Talk

Listen to your self-talk. Many times we heap up more stress by negative and blaming self-talk. Begin to genuinely tune in and listen to how you are talking to yourself. As you take note of a thought, if it's negative simply reverse it. You may be thinking, "I will never make that deadline…."

Simply turn that around and think, "I will do my level best to make that deadline and that's all anyone can do."

Needed Sleep

Sleep deprivation is yet another thing that adds to stress levels. A deep, healthy sleep is necessary for the body to restore itself. Those who fail to understand the need for a good night's sleep think nothing of staying up until all hours of the night – often just watching television.

To work with Michael Von Irvin or make comments contact
help@writersprofitguide.com

Take the necessary steps to prepare in the evening for quieting your mind and body. If the evening news sets your nerves on edge, then stop watching it. If the bills are piling up, handle them during the day rather than right before going to sleep. In other words, lessen the stress load before bedtime. Determine that you will begin to treat your sleep as a priority rather than a luxury.

If you have been following the directives that have been presented in the previous chapters of this book, then you are already improving your chances of enjoying a good night sleep. Because of your better food choices, no longer will you lie awake suffering from indigestion. With regard to regular exercise, studies have shown that exercise helps a person sleep sounder and longer, and then feel more awake during the day.

Stress levels can be controlled. Make it your goal to learn as many stress-relieving techniques as you possibly can and then begin incorporating them into the routine of your daily life. Then watch how your newly relaxed body can begin to successfully deal with symptoms related to prediabetes and diabetes.

Conclusion

In the introduction, this statistic was given:

25.8 million Americans have diabetes — 8.3 percent of the U.S. population. Of these, 7 million do not know they have the disease.

Where are you in this statistic? You need to know. Not only do you need to know, you also need to take action now to protect yourself from ever becoming one of those 25.8 million people who have diabetes.

Over and over again medical experts state that not only is diabetes preventable, it is also *reversible*. This is news that should give hope to a great many people.

To work with Michael Von Irvin or make comments contact
help@writersprofitguide.com

By reading ***The No Hogwash Approach to Understanding Diabetes***, you have learned how intricately your body is designed. All parts of your body work together like a highly-tuned machine. This is why one prescription, or one fat diet, or a membership to the local gym is not the answer. Instead seek to support every single system and organ of your body. You can do this by eating nutrient-rich food, by moving your body with a good exercise program, and dealing with stress rather than becoming a victim of it.

These are just a few ways to move toward optimum health. But if you will determine to start with these, you will be miles down the road toward your goal.

Good luck and good health.

www.michaelvonirvin.com

Made in the USA
Middletown, DE
12 April 2019